Meno Estradiol – A Medical Guide

(All References Included)

By Dan Purser MD

Explained & Discussed in this book:

- Estrogen Dominance
- Proper Estrogen Replacement
- Estradiol Options & Prescriptions
- Estrogen Window or Ten Year Window
- Osteoporosis Prescriptions & Benefits
- DVT & Blood Clot Risks
- Current Research & Articles Referenced

© 2016 by Dan Purser MD and DP Publishing

All Rights Reserved. No part of this publication may be reproduced in any form or by any means, including scanning, photocopying, or otherwise without prior written permission of the copyright holder.

First Printing, 2016-09-01

Printed in the United States of America

Preface

Menopause, Estrogen, And Estradiol – A Medical Guide

Explained & Discussed in this book:

- Estrogen Dominance
- Proper Estrogen Replacement
- Estradiol Options & Prescriptions
- Estrogen Window or Ten Year Window
- Osteoporosis Prescriptions & Benefits
- DVT & Blood Clot Risks
- Current Research & Articles Referenced

There's a lot of confusion around using estrogens or estradiol in menopause (pre or post) and this little highly referenced book tries to cut through all the confusion to give you answers, and show you results.

I discuss osteoporosis, estradiol, vaginal atrophy, skin wrinkles, DVT, blood clots, pulmonary embolism, and breast cancer. I give you this in laymen's terms. I tell you what I'd want you to know as my patient.

Menopause, Estrogen, And Estradiol says it all – the good and the bad.

So find out why I've had 13 #1 books on Amazon, two in the Amazon Top 100 so far this year alone. I've also had the top medical book on Amazon for a month in this summer

(2016). And I am ranked as one of the Top Medical Authors on Amazon.

This is just a little gem for those who think or wonder if they might need estradiol.

Thanks for buying Menopause, Estrogens, And Estradiol. Good luck and STAY HEALTHY.

Disclaimers

Income Disclaimer

This document contains business strategies, marketing methods and other business advice that, regardless of my own results and experience, may not produce the same results (or any results) for you. I make absolutely no guarantee, expressed or implied, that by following the advice below you will make any money or improve current profits, as there are several factors and variables that come into play regarding any given business.

Primarily, results will depend on the nature of the product or medication used, the conditions of the marketplace, the past and current medical history and condition of the patient, the experience of the individual, and situations and elements that are beyond your control.

As with any educational advice, you assume all risks related to thearpy or treatments based on your own discretion and at your own potential expense.

Liability Disclaimer

By reading this document, you assume all risks associated with using the advice given below, with a full understanding that you, solely, are responsible for anything that may occur as a result of putting this information into action in any way, and regardless of your interpretation of the advice.

You further agree that our company cannot be held responsible in any way for the success or failure of your business as a result of the information presented below. It is your responsibility to conduct your own due diligence regarding the safe and successful operation of your business if you intend to apply any of our information in any way to your business operations.

Terms of Use

You are given a non-transferable, "personal use" license to this product. You cannot distribute it or share it with other individuals.

Also, there are no resale rights or private label rights granted when purchasing this document. In other words, it's for your own personal use only.

Foreword

This book is my attempt to strike at the roots of ignorance when it comes to estradiol.

Bizarrely, even my mentioning estradiol usage to many doctors is a controversial thing, so in polite company I tend to leave it unmentioned. But I've been asked to speak about women's hormones and natural hormone replacement therapies all over the world, because when we're all of the same race—we're all humans—we realize, every woman needs estrogens.

This book is about the natural estrogen which your ovaries produce – ESTRADIOL – mostly, and some about estriol. This is touchy stuff, so I had to put in all the references – I don't want any lawsuits based on what I wrote. So make sure your doctor also approves before you use estrogens. They need to have done their own research and not just followed mine.

I am talking about 17β-estradiol here, the exact substance your ovaries leak out and produce most of your adult life.

No studies have shown estradiol is harmful if used correctly, in fact it's been found to be incredibly beneficial if used properly, and its use is associated with a decrease in breast cancer, not an increase.

I hope this little book helps you in some way.

This book is directly connected to its companion course Estradiol for Menopause. Go to danpursermd.com and hover over the "For Women" tab and and then click the Menopause Video Courses.

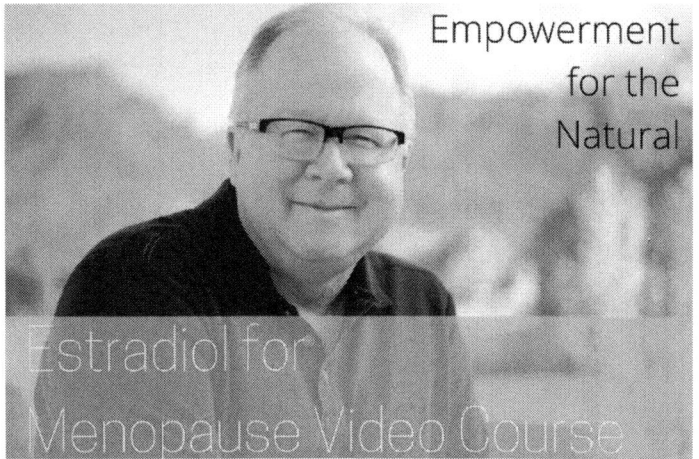

Table of Contents

Chapter 1 11
The Hormonal or Neuroendocrine Theory of Aging

Chapter 2 13
Flawed HRT Studies That Ruined HRT For Everybody?

Chapter 3 18
History Questions – Start Here Before You See Your Doctor

Chapter 4 21
Erroneous Beliefs That Must Be Understood & Dispelled

Chapter 5 24
Estrogen (Usually Estradiol and Estriol) Prescribing

Chapter 6 27
Effects Of No Estrogen?

Chapter 7 28
Six Reasons Not To Take Post-Menopausal Oral Estradiol

Chapter 8 29
Natural Estradiol Use In Osteoporosis

Chapter 9 33
Estradiol In Vaginal Atrophy

Chapter 10 35
Tips, Pointers and Clary Sage

Chapter 1

The Hormonal or Neuroendocrine Theory of Aging

Let's start with a little history.

First proposed by Professor Vladimir Dilman and Ward Dean MD, the hormonal theory elaborates on aging by focusing on the neuroendocrine system[1]. This system is a network of biochemicals that govern the release of hormones which are altered by the gland called the hypothalamus located in the brain. The hypothalamus controls various feedback mechanisms to instruct other organs and glands to release their hormones. The hypothalamus, acting as a master gland, also responds to the body hormone levels as a guide to the overall hormonal activity. As we grow older, the hypothalamus loses its precision regulatory ability and the receptors which uptake individual hormones become less sensitive to them (thyroid receptors in the periphery, for example).

Accordingly as we age, the secretion of many hormones declines, and their effectiveness (compared unit to unit) is also reduced due to the receptors becoming less functional (each cell in your body has hundreds, if not thousands, of receptors each designed to handle a specific hormone.

One theory for the hypothalamus loss of regulation is that it is damaged by the hormone cortisol. Cortisol is produced from the adrenal glands (located on the kidneys), and cortisol is considered to be a dark-hormone responsible for stress. It is known to be one of the few hormones that increase with age. As discussed in other chapters in this book, the effects of cortisol floating around in your body can be offset by nutriceutically available hormones such as melatonin, or adaptogens (various herbs that lower cortisol and improve response to stress).

If cortisol damages the hypothalamus, then over time this becomes a downward spiral of continued hypothalamic damage, leading to an ever increasing degree of cortisol production, and thus more hypothalamic damage.

This damage could then lead to hormonal imbalance as the hypothalamus loses its ability to control the system. Such an argument demands the use of cortisol adjusters (such as DHEA, or phenytoin) or adaptogens to help slow down the cortisol accumulation. The decline in the functional capability of peripheral receptors can be partially offset by receptor resensitizers such as the drug metformin (which improves insulin sensitivity by assiting the insulin receptor – another hormone receptor).

So to prevent aging, to keep us in that young, healthy, rich hormonal milieu where we had so much fun and optimal health, we need hormones that are biologically identical to those we humans produce in our own bodies and in the proper amounts that are reflected in the levels we lived with while we were in our prime (age 25-32). The medical research literature is replete with studies and articles in support of these positions and we'll delve into these as we move forward.

Chapter 2
Flawed HRT Studies That Ruined HRT For Everybody?

This is a list of key studies that are critical to the understanding of this book and the current dynamics involving prescribing or suggesting the use of estradiol or estrogens for menopause.

HERS (Heart and Estrogen/progestin Replacement Study[2]): Participants were postmenopausal women with previously diagnosed CHD who were randomly assigned to receive conjugated equine estrogens and medroxyprogesterone, or identical placebo and then followed-up for an average of 4.1 years. The conclusion was that hormone therapy had no overall effect on CHD risk in the HERS trial, despite the expected favorable effects on HDL and LDL-C levels. The real outcome though has been the systematic horrification of millions of women and their physicians worldwide, and the resulting fear and trepidation to using or taking any female hormones, and synthetic side effect intensive hormones being erroneously discussed in the popular and medical press as if they were real human hormones.

For example, as reported by Denise Grady in the February 6, 2001 edition of **The New York Times®** in her article titled **A New Look At Estrogen And Stroke[3]**, she discusses the HERS study as reported in **Circulation®** and concluded that women with heart disease cannot assume hormone replacement therapy will protect them from stroke. In her explanation she did not differentiate between the synthetic progestational agent/equine conjugated estrones combination used in the study and actual human hormones that were available then and are still.

If you're really interested (or a physician), see the flip side of this argument (my side) – see the 1995 article **Menopause®** in **The Medical Clinics of North America®** by Joel Hargrove, M.D.[4] who was chair of the Menopause Clinics at Vanderbilt University School of Medicine. **WHI (Women's Health Initiative Postmenopausal Hormone Therapy Trials[5]):** This is the Study that we've all heard so much about. Created by the National Institutes of Health (NIH)®– specifically, the National Heart, Lung and Blood Institute (NHLBI)® this study was designed to define the risks and benefits of interventions, notably hormone therapy, to potentially prevent heart disease, breast and colorectal cancer, and osteoporotic fractures in postmenopausal women. On the basis of results from this study and their interpretation by the lead investigators, "guidelines for the use of hormone therapy in postmenopausal women changed. For the study as a whole...161,809 women aged 50 to 79 years were enrolled in either an observational study or clinical trials of low dietary fat vs. self-selected diet, estrogen and progesterone therapy (HT) or estrogen therapy alone (ET) vs. placebo, or calcium and vitamin D supplementation vs. placebo."

Wait... Huh? What? This study used estrogen and progesterone? Really? Naah, not really! Read on...

"The larger of the 2 studies evaluating postmenopausal hormone therapy randomized nonhysterectomized women to estrogen plus progestin (0.625 mg conjugated **equine** estrogens [CEE] + 2.5 mg medroxyprogesterone acetate (MPA), Prempro®, N = 8506 women) or placebo (N = 8102 women). Monitoring of these subjects began in the fall of

1997 and was scheduled to last until 2005.

However, the Data Safety Monitoring Board® (DSMB) terminated the HT arm of the WHI early when a predetermined threshold of excess cases of breast cancer was reached.[6] The smaller hormone study involved 10,739 women who had undergone hysterectomy; they were randomized to receive estrogen alone (0.625 CEE, Premarin®) or placebo. The ET arm was terminated March 2, 2004 -- also early -- because of increased risk of stroke."

Let us clarify here and now . . .

MEDROXYPROGESTERONE and CONJUGATED EQUINE ESTRONES are NOT human hormones!

Human serum medroxyprogesterone levels are not even measurable! And they exposed 161,809 women to this FDA approved big money-making patented drug?

Let's see what the press had to say – surely they caught this study error...

As reported by Leslie Berger in the June 6, 2004 edition of **The New York Times®** in her article titled TWO YEARS AFTER; **On Hormone Therapy, the Dust Is Still Settling**[7] where she notes that two years after the bombshell results of the WHI was dropped on hormone replacement therapy, there were at that time signs that the rush away from the drugs was finally ending. She then goes on to note that how in July 2002, a federal study, part of the Women's Health Initiative, was halted when its data showed the dangers of hormone therapy outweighing its long-term benefits.

After the study, sales of the drugs -- estrogen and estrogen-progestin – plunged.

Well, this article is a little better – they called it progestin this time but still did not mention human hormones, nor did they really differentiate between progestins (synthetic) and progesterone (human hormone).

Or how about this most recent study on HRT and breast cancer?

The Million Women Study?

Let's look at the abstract in Pub Med® by Reeves GK, et al. (For the Million Women Study Collaborators. Cancer Research UK Epidemiology Unit, University of Oxford, UK. Hormonal therapy for menopause and breast-cancer risk by histological type: a cohort study and metaanalysis. Lancet Oncol. 2006 Nov;7(11):910-8.).[8] There is no mention in this abstract (we presume it's written by health care professionals) as to the kind of hormones actually used (synthetics and nonhuman hormones: equine conjugated estrogens and progestogens). You as a potential patient or your doctor as a professional are then left assuming that all hormone replacement therapies are going to cause some level of breast cancer, when the literature, as we are about to detail, is replete with completely opposite observations.

To further buttress the natural position on HRT, know the European medical community looks at us in the USA more than a little askance for our weird and confusing opinions in this country (and by those who should know better) in a 2003 **Maturitas** Critical Comment[9]:

"In the paper, the Authors confuse ethinyl estradiol with 17-β-estradiol."

This is a HUGE error in the Million Women Study since they blame real human 17-β-estradiol with causing breast cancer when it's a well known and highly researched fact that CEE (ethinyl estradiol) causes breast cancer (while 17-β-estradiol appears to lead to a decrease in breast cancer risk of 30%). Yet the anti-HRT crew went nuts (and still are) with this study and its spin offs – all wrong in regards to safety and the use of estradiol in menopause.

This is the misinformation storm you, your doctor, and I fight against every day when we try to make safe and educated choices to treat you.

Chapter 3

History Questions – Start Here Before You See Your Doctor

Do you really want or need estrogens or estradiol?

Start with asking yourself these questions before going to talk to your doctor.

Female Hormonal History Questions

1. Are you concerned about facial skin wrinkles? Other skin wrinkles?

2. Are you concerned about depression? Do you ever feel blue?

3. Are you concerned about improving your sex life?

4. Are you concerned about keeping strong?

5. Are you concerned about keeping fit?

6. Are you concerned about healthy bones?

7. Have you ever been told you have osteoporosis?

8. Any family history of osteoporosis?

9. Have you been through menopause?

10. When did your mother go through menopause?

11. What are your periods like?

12. How many pregnancies have you had? How many deliveries?

13. Any complications of delivery? Post-partum hemorrhaging?

14. Do you ever have sexual problems?

15. Ever have difficulty getting sexually aroused?

16. Ever feel breathless?

17. Are you concerned about memory loss? Do you have any memory loss?

18. Do you ever lose your way while driving or shopping?

19. Are you concerned about increased weight?

20. Have you gained weight lately or in the last few years? If so, how much?

21. Are you concerned about decreased libido (decreased sex drive)?

22. Are you concerned about dry eyes, or dry skin, or a dry vagina?

23. Are you concerned about tooth loss?

24. Do you ever feel fatigue?

25. Are you concerned about your genitalia drying and shriveling up?

26. Are you concerned about reducing your risk of heart disease?

27. Do you drink alcohol? How much?

28. Do you take narcotics? How often? Which ones?

29. Have you had painful joints or been diagnosed with osteoarthritis?

30. Have you ever had breast, ovarian, or uterine/cervical cancer?

Chapter 4

Erroneous Beliefs That Must Be Understood & Dispelled

With the reporting of HERS[10] and WHI[181] studies, hormone replacement therapy (HRT) has been saddled with several erroneous beliefs that we will quickly explode. Then it is our hope that you will consider the much more physiological and natural approach of replacement therapy with modern biologically identical human hormones.

HRT Erroneous Belief #1

"Estrogen and progesterone were the hormones used in those studies and they're bad for me, right doctor? They cause cancer, heart attacks, and strokes, right?"

Wrong, AND right.

Estrogen and progesterone as created in the human body – natural estrogens and progesterones – were **not** used in either of those studies. Synthetic progestational agents that are foreign to your body, and very inflammatory for your blood vessels and heart were used in both studies as were conjugated equine estrogen -- taken from pregnant mare's urine – another problematic hormone substance for human females. Both of these have been proven to be injurious when given long term before these studies, so smarter physicians in general are not sure why they were used in these important studies.

Conjugated equine estrogen (Premarin®), used in both studies, contains some estradiol and some estriol (which partially converts to estrone in the human body), but contains other hormones that are not conducive to long term women's health – there lies the problem.

HRT Erroneous Belief #2

"So, doctor, if you won't give me those hormones because they're so bad (not that I would let you any way), then what do you suggest?"

Good question.

For more than a decade, there have been widely available in this country biologically identical human hormones that give you excellent benefits with minimal effects when given properly. Levels can be tracked with blood tests (which cannot be done with synthetic progestational agents), and adjusted accordingly. These hormones are identical to what every woman makes in their bodies.

HRT Erroneous Belief #3

"But doesn't estrogen cause breast cancer?"

The conjugated equine estrogens in Premarin® contain carcinogenic equilin and equilenin, which can cause breast cancer (the 17 alpha-dihydroderivatives of equilenin and equilin -- 15% of the CEE components -- have a non-estrogenic or even an anti-estrogenic effect on breast tissue).[11]

On the other hand, biologically identical human estrogens have not been associated in any studies with breast cancer. Regardless, estrogens should always be properly opposed with human progesterone.

HRT Erroneous Belief #4

"So taking Premarin® won't give me any human estrogens? Wouldn't a natural estrogen be better?"

Not true. Patients who take Premarin® almost always have levels beyond these therapeutic levels when randomly checked.

The trouble with conjugated equine estrones is what they carry with them – equilin and equilenin and their derivatives, which are associated with breast cancer and exaggerated potency in the hepatic system.[12] But if a choice had to be made, Premarin® is far superior to no estrogens at all because of concentration and estrogen load.

Chapter 5

Estrogen (Usually Estradiol and Estriol) Prescribing

(Note: Only for surgical or FSH-elevated (>50 mIU/ml[13]) confirmed menopause.)

Human estrogen is produced in four different forms[14] – estrone (E1), estradiol (E2), estriol (E3), and estetrol (E4 -- 15α-hydroxyestriol -- in pregnancy only). Estradiol is the most physiologically and biologically active, and the one which offers the most protection and benefits. It also converts to estrone which, along with estradiol, also converts to estriol, so technically and theoretically (if the patient is young enough to have all their CYP3A7 cytochrome P-450 16-hydroxylation liver conversion enzymes remaining intact[15]) it can be the only estrogen you need to give. But usually this form of HRT is given orally or transdermally (only in certain situations) as a bi-estrogen, or BiEst, containing both estradiol and estriol (many people believe that estriol protects against cancer, but there have been no studies to prove this) or more specifically human 17-β-estradiol which can also be given in a compounded form or as Estrace® (or generic estradiol) at 1 mgm a day, which usually gives high enough levels to provide proper cardiovascular protection[16].

Dosing and Manner

ORAL

The estradiol can be compounded in a capsule, or given as a generic or big pharma version (Estrace®). Most often it should be given orally as 17-β-estradiol (E2) at either 1.0-2.0 mgm or as Estrace® 1.0 mgm orally a day. The estradiol level can be raised to 1.5 mgm, or 2.0 mgm or decreased to 0.5 mgm (you can choose not to give the estriol for a number of good reasons).

Note that estriol (E3) is the breakdown product of estradiol (E2), and because of this does not actually have to be given.

CREAMS

Estrace® does come in a cream or as a generic cream at 1.0 mg/gram (or as a compounded as a cream). There are only a few situations in which I choose to use the cream:

1. if a woman is past the Ten Year Window (10 years past menopause without having ever taken oral estradiol)[17], or

2. if they have had clots or DVTs (deep venous thromboses), the potential (such as post-menopausal hypertension) for a pro-thrombotic mutation (i.e. a clotting disorder) or Factor V Leiden, or

3. if I wish to use it for vaginal dryness or atrophy along with compounded testosterone cream.

(NOTE: CRITICAL: If a woman is past the Ten Year Window -- 10 years past menopause without having ever taken any form of oral estradiol. IF past this window then they have a *high risk of a heart attack or stroke* if they suddenly start ORAL estradiol. This is due to the first pass effect that occurs in the liver with oral estradiol, which in turn causes metallothioneins to form that break plaque loose in carotid and cardiac arteries.)

PATCHES

Estrace® comes in a patch or as a generic patch – I tend to use the 0.1 mg/day patch (the largest one) because I offset it with natural progesterone (see my #1 Best Selling Amazon "Top 100" book *PROGESTERONE: The Women's Ultimate Feel Good Hormone*) in order to get the best kevelks (again >50 mIU/ml). There are only a few situations in which I choose to use the patches:

1. if a woman is past the Ten Year Window, or

2. if they have had clots or DVTs (deep venous thromboses), the potential (such as post-menopausal hypertension) for a pro-thrombotic mutation (i.e. a clotting disorder) or Factor V Leiden.

HOW TO TAKE?

(Oral vs Topical → Oral estradiol gives the best cardiovascular protection.) *[Use ONLY 17β-Estradio,1 as it's bio-identical. I don't use bi-est or tri-est.]* "oral estrogen offers more cardiovascular benefits." "many studies claim transdermal estrogen does **not** provide any cardiovascular protection." "because **oral estrogen passes through the liver to improve cholesterol health**. Since transdermal estrogen bypasses the liver to directly enter the bloodstream, it cannot provide advantageous lipid effects." [18]

Chapter 6
Effects Of No Estrogen?

1. Vaginal atrophy (though this occurs more so from lack of testosterone)
2. Urinary incontinence
3. Hot flashes
4. Temperature dysregulation
5. Balance problems
6. Sagging skin -- transdermal estriol helps this
7. Sagging breasts
8. Epidermal thinning, declining dermal collagen content, diminished skin moisture, decreased laxity, and impaired wound healing
9. Fatigue
10. Depression
11. Mood swings
12. Declining libido to no libido
13. Acceleration of glomerulosclerosis (scarring in the kidney)
14. Osteoporosis
15. Coronary artery disease -- the #1 reason to take estradiol
16. Sexual dysfunction
17. Tooth loss and receding gums (always attractive)

Chapter 7

Six Reasons Not To Take Post-Menopausal <u>Oral</u> Estradiol

(Even though oral is usually more beneficial.)

1. Your doctor said not to (for whatever reason).

2. You've had estrogen receptor positive (ER+) breast or ovarian cancer.

3. You don't have progesterone to take to oppose it (always oppose estrogen with natural progesterone).

4. You have Factor V Leiden and/or any other clotting disorders (you can only use topical progesterone – ONLY).

5. You have post-menopausal hypertension (high blood pressure), treated or not (11X increased risk of a pro-thrombotic mutation – See #4[19]).

6. You're outside the "10 Year Window".

Chapter 8

Natural Estradiol Use In Osteoporosis

Fractures from osteoporosis are a major killer of elderly women, and it's our fault if we let one of our patients get so osteoporotic that they fracture something and die. We are generally NOT doing a very good job of preventing this.[20]

For a more detailed explanation, please refer to my best selling book **Resolving Osteoporosis: The Cure & Guide Book** available on Amazon and iBooks.

It's our fault if they need Fosamax®, too. If this occurs, we have not handled these patients appropriately.

Sadly, 54 % of women have osteopenia, 30 % have osteoporosis. 97% of free living women >71 years of age and 99% of nursing home women have a Vitamin D deficiency.[21]

Diagnosis of Osteoporosis: Get baseline dual-energy x-ray absorptiometry[22] (DeXA which is the gold standard for measuring bone density) to diagnose. Repeat the BMD (DeXA) every two years (that's how fast it changes and how often Medicare will pay for it).

Get a NTX test (2nd urine of the morning) to track more effectively (changes within a few months).[23] Patients can get this annually. NTX tells you if there's immediate ongoing loss or gain of bone mineral density (BMD).

Check estradiol[24] and progesterone levels, too.

You can also get the main circulating Vitamin D3 levels

(25 OHD or 25–Hydroxy-Vitamin D).[25]

Calcium levels (other than intracellular via a Spectracell®) are not helpful, while knowing their average daily calcium dose is (should be 1500 mg premenopause and 1000 mg per day postmenopause.)

Treatment of Osteoporosis:

Vitamin D3 (cholecalciferol) is more potent than D2 (ergocalciferol): It improves osteoporosis.[26]

D3 decreases fall risk.

Vitamin K2 is more potent than K1: It promotes the synthesis of proteins involved with calcium utilization, increases absorption of calcium from the gut, and decreases fracture risk.[27]

Both Sexes > 65 yrs of age:

For physicians: Use Alendronate (Fosamax®) EVERY time[28] just to protect you from lawsuits, etc. Although biphosphonates have been shown to reduce bone resorption and inhibit osteoclasts, their effectiveness seems to be best for treatment in women with osteoporosis, and they do not appear to work as well as estrogens in prevention of osteoporosis.[29] Although Quandt and colleagues[30] have found that alendronate therapy in women with osteopenia reduces vertebral fracture risk, Schousboe and colleagues performed a cost-effectiveness analysis to estimate the cost per quality-adjusted life-year (QALY) gained from a five-year alendronate (Fosamax) regimen in women 55 to 75 years of age with osteopenia and no additional risk factors, the final result suggesting that it costs more than a reasonable amount.[31]

Let us restate that – alendronate is not cost effective to use.

Ibandronate (Boniva®) is a biphosphonate that can be taken daily or monthly. The daily dosage has been shown to decrease vertebral fractures in women with osteoporosis and a history of previous vertebral fractures. It has not been shown to reduce the risk of hip fracture or other nonvertebral fracture, nor to reduce fractures in women without prior fracture. Ibandronate has not been compared directly with other bisphosphonates, or with adequate daily doses of calcium and vitamin D.[32]

Let us restate that – alendronate and ibandronate just reduce the incidence of fractures and reduce the bone loss BUT they do not increase the BMD – they just slow the rate of loss and are not cost effective (unlike HRT and Vitamin D/Cal Mag Aspartate).

As a matter of fact, no biphosphonate has been compared with adequate doses of calcium and vitamin D[33][34] which we know are inexpensive, side effect free (actually taking adequate doses of either gives you a huge list of benefits), and very effective[35] in combination.

Biphosphonates have been shown to slow the demineralization of patient's bones, but studies have not clearly shown that biphosphonates reverse bone loss – unlike hormones![36] **(Read the studies!)** HRT is much cheaper and more effective than alendronate according to the experts! Do your job, physicians!

But to prevent easy malpractice suits, put every osteoporotic patient you have on Fosamax®, because even the attorneys won't understand what we just said.

Understand?

*Oral Estradiol with appropriate optimized serum levels prevents, improves, and even reverses osteopenia and osteoporosis.[37] Also, it can improve muscle strength and decrease fall risk[38] (again important). This is the same with Vitamin D3!

*Take Calcium with Magnesium in a Cal-Mag combination at 2–5 pills per day[39] to reduce osteopenia/-porosis. This combination also reduces hsCRP.

*Vitamin D3 (800-1000 IU/day) with Vitamin K1 [or Phytonadione] (100 mcg/day) or

K2 [Menaquinone] 45-90 mcg/day).[40]

*All calcium carbonate contains high lead levels, so use a Calcium Citrate or Cal-Mag Aspartat supplement.[41]

*For optimal Zinc and Magnesium and safety, take a better vitamin, but one with no iron[42] and no copper[43] (very hard to find) – these act as very detrimental pro-oxidants, especially in people over 40.

*Increased fruits and vegetables (i.e. as in the DASH diet) reduce osteoporosis.[44]

*Take B12/Folate to reduce homocysteine levels -- lower homocysteine levels reduce fracture risk, too.[45]

Chapter 9

Estradiol In Vaginal Atrophy

Vaginal Atrophy (One More Time)

Vaginal atrophy is far easier to prevent than to treat, but if you wish to treat it effectively make sure your patient's level of testosterone is adequate, as this seems to be the best way to promote vaginal moisture and can even cause a slight discharge (please tell your patients to wear a pad if this becomes annoying, as too much moisture is far superior and healthier than having the Sahara Desert down there). This urogenital atrophy can also lead to a decline in sexual desire and functionality, so take testosterone cream.[46]

Second, if the oral estrogen is not working then add a local estrogen[47] (according to their histories and needs) such as:

PREFERRED (if you are also giving oral E2) -- Estring® -- ONLY localized levels of estrogen, so it gives vaginal protection only!

Femring® -- Increases circulating levels of estrogen, so vaginal/osteoporosis protection in provided.

Vagifem® tablets – Increases circulating levels of estrogen, so vaginal/osteoporosis protection is provided.

Note that these avoid the FIRST PASS EFFECT in the liver, and so do not effect lipids or give cardioprotection as effectively as oral estradiol. If you are at risk for heart disease, take the oral estradiol if it's safe (i.e. if they are not past the window[48] and have no hypertension [Prothrombin variant[49]])!

Preventing vaginal atrophy prevents stress incontinence, too.

Note that this vaginal or urogenital atrophy can lead to stress incontinence which is, as we've said, a LOT easier to prevent than to treat, once it occurs. If this is starting to occur in you, push the estradiol levels a little higher OR add the local estradiol rings or tablets to prevent this problem.

Chapter 10

Tips, Pointers and Clary Sage

Here are my tips and pointers for physicians and patients (public). Hope they help.

If premenopausal or perimenopausal or even premenstrual syndrome (all the kinds of PMS out there) give them 100-200 mgm progesterone triturates for sublingual dissolution whenever they start to have these symptoms. Help them!

If you get these symptoms in someone who is postmenopausal and on modern HRT, and increasing their progesterone does not work, lower the dose of estradiol you are giving.

Practice Gems on Estrogen Supplementation

1. Protect your patient from cancers, cataracts and heart disease – it is your obligation –give them proper HRT protection.

2. Give them Estrace® 1 mg a day if their insurance will cover it. Give them generic Estrace® if they are financially struggling and have no insurance. (At Walmart® on their $10 list; it's even cheaper at Costco®.)

3. Ask your patients if they want to be dried up like a prune and have incredibly wrinkled skin, no teeth, and no sex – or

would they like some estrogen?

4. Pre-/Perimenopausal Situations: look at FSH levels which porpoise (go up and down). If your patient is premenopausal, you can give progesterone only (1 to 12 tablets a day) –they make plenty of estrogen naturally. No use checking levels of estradiol or progesterone in these patients. If perimenopausal, check FSH levels, and if high then treat, if they are low, you can use progesterone – there's no harm in giving progesterone to an anovulatory perimenopausal woman. If they want to have a heavier menstration (ask them) just stop the progesterone – if they don't want to, continue the progesterone. After 3 to 6 months stop the progesterone, after one month check a FSH level to see where they are.

5. It does you no good to measure pre-menopausal estradiol and progesterone levels, because you don't know where your patients are in their cycle. Check FSH and LH levels instead if you are so concerned.

6. You can diagnose menopause by symptoms – if your patient experiences no menses for six months, it's menopause. This goes for almost any age, any symptoms. If they request treatment, you better suspect menopause. Measure the FSH and LH (if both are >50 this is an indication of menopause).

7. Use human biologically identical hormones, not equine urine estrones which (i.e. CEE as we've said repeatedly) contain seventeen androgenic and carcinogenic agents.

8. Do not use estrone. It is not breast tissue friendly. This is also already created in the stomach lining to such an extent that most women are never short of estrone.

9. If you have a patient on HRT, aggressively communicate the need for PAP and breast mammograms – every 2 years

according to the American Cancer Association and ACOG (if they are past age 40), but annually, if possible. Send out letters. Do everything possible for them to get checked.

MALPRACTICE WARNING: Do not refill HRT unless they comply!

10. Don't guess. If you really have no idea, then check the levels! Optimal estradiol level is 50-100 ng/ml. You can get annoying side effects if above 100 (breast tenderness, vaginal bleeding, bloating, breaking out), but must be at least 50 ng/ml to give protection.

11. There is no need to cycle estradiol after menopause – give it every day!

12. If your patient has had their uterus and ovaries removed, and doesn't have a breast cancer risk factor, then give them everything – Estradiol, Testosterone, DHEA, and Progesterone. Save their lives!

13. MALPRACTICE WARNING: Absolute contraindications – unresolved history of clots, thrombosis, emboli, or HTN (hypertension). DO NOT GIVE THESE PATIENTS ORAL ESTROGEN! Give them an estradiol patch (Climara®) or an estrogen ring (see below). (Note: the patch does not help as strongly against CV disease[50] as oral.)

14. If your patient has hot flashes that are not resolved with progesterone, go to BID with the Estrace® for 6 months or so until the symptoms resolve.

15. If your patient doesn't have hot flashes until after you start the BiEst (or estradiol), then double the dose for 6 months or so, but if this does not resolve the hot flashes then switch them to a topical patch such as Climara® or Yasmin® (the least androgenic BCPs on the market and for

that reason, as this book is written) as BCP can also decrease hot flashes, so try if you're desperate. Know, though, that hot flashes are actually usually caused by perimenopausal decline of the hormone inhibin.[51]

The other opinion, in regards to hot flashes, is that in some women catecholestrogens (estrogen metabolites) are caused from oral estrogen[52]. In essence, "resetting the thermostat" is to blame for the hot flashes[53] – if you suspect this is the case switch your patients to the Climara® patch for great 24 hour coverage – it's worth a try.

16. Be aware that (very rarely) patients can start ovulating on the natural hormones and can get pregnant – warn them if they are younger postmenopausal patients (especially with menopause secondary to pituitary damage)!!!

17. If the patient is past the window for HRT (age 50-60 years), or has hypertension (thus a prothrombotic risk), use a vaginal estradiol ring or tablet. Femring® and Vagifem® tablets give proper estradiol levels similar to the Climara® patch, while Estring® is for those women with breast cancer, DVT, or MI histories who are having localized vaginal issues (urinary frequency, dry vagina, incontinence, etc) and in who you do not want circulating estrogens. The Femring®/Vagifem® option can treat hot flashes in some patients (in the occasional instances when progesterone does not).

18. Warning! Estriol (E3) tends to cause bloating or the feeling of bloating and if this occurs among your HRT patients, stop their estriol first. Give a diuretic next (i.e. Dyazide®).

There is absolutely no need to check estradiol levels in men. What is being said on the internet is WRONG! If true, at what level would they like the estradiol level to rise before intervention with anastrozole is begun? There is no answer to this, because Estradiol is cardioprotective and prevents strokes in men.[54] Leave it alone unless they get significant breast enlargement!

Now that you're aware of the benefits of estradiol and why you'd want to keep normal levels after menopause, let's look at an oil or two that can support your levels.

Lavender

History of Lavender

The use of lavender has been recorded for more than 2,500 years. Egyptians, Phoenicians and the people of Arabia used lavender as a perfume -- and also for mummification, by wrapping the dead in lavender-dipped shrouds. In ancient Greece, lavender was called "nardus," "nard," or "spikenard" (named for the Syrian city of Naarda) and was used as a cure for everything from insomnia and aching backs to insanity.

By Roman times, lavender had already become a prized commodity. Lavender flowers were sold to ancient Romans for 100 denarii per pound -- equivalent to a full month's wage for a farm laborer -- and were used to scent the water in Roman baths. In fact, the baths served as the root of the plant's current name. "Lavender" is derived from the Latin lavare, meaning, "to wash." Romans also used lavender as a perfume, insect repellent and flavoring. They even added dried lavender into their smoking mixtures.

In Medieval and Renaissance Europe, lavender was strewn over the stone floors of castles to be used as a disinfectant and deodorant. It was also one of many medicinal herbs grown in "infirmarian's gardens," with yields intended to be used to ward off disease. Use of lavender was highly revered during the Great Plague of London in the 17th century, when individuals fastened bunches of lavender to each wrist to protect themselves from the Black Death. Glove makers scented their stocks of leather with lavender oil to ward off the disease. Thieves who made a living stealing from the graves and the homes of Plague victims concocted a wash known as "Four Thieves Vinegar," which contained lavender, to cleanse and protect themselves after a night's work. Today, we know the disease was transmitted by fleas, so the use of lavender--which is known to repel these insects -- could very well have saved lives and prevented further spread of the plague.

The Shakers, a strict sect of English Quakers, are credited with commercializing lavender and introducing a variety of lavender-based products to the United States and Canada. The Shakers raised their own herbs, produced medicines, and sold them to neighbors and customers outside their religious sect. Because the Shakers believed in celibacy, they probably did not explore the romantic, sensual appeal that lavender is said to have, but there are many others throughout history who have, including Cleopatra, who, according to legend, used lavender to seduce Julius Caesar and Mark Antony.

Medicinal, Therapeutic & Practical Uses

Lavender is grown commercially for extraction of its oil from its flowers and to some degree from its foliage. The oil is obtained through a distillation process.

The oil is used as a disinfectant, an antiseptic, an anti-inflammatory and for aromatherapy. An infusion of Lavender is claimed to soothe and heal insect bites, sunburns, small cuts, burns and inflammatory conditions and even acne. Lavender oils are also used for internal medical conditions, among others indigestion and heartburn.

Lavender oil is said to soothe headaches, migraines and motion sickness when applied to the temples. It is frequently used as an aid to sleep and relaxation.

Dried Lavender flowers are used extensively as fragrant herbal filler inside sachets - to freshen linens, closets and drawers. As an air spray, it is used to freshen practically any room. Dried lavender flowers have also become popular at weddings as decorations, gifts and as confetti for tossing over the newlyweds.

Why am I discussing Lavender?

Beacause it is believed to contain sclareol (more on this below) – not much is but some – as a matter of fact, it is somewhat similar to clary sage.

Studies have shown lavender essential oil to also be estrogenic – just miniamally though. And the data seemed anecdotal at best. But it's cousin, clary sage, is a whole different story.

Clary Sage

History of Clary Sage

"The Romans called it sclarea, from claurus, or "clear," because they used it as an eyewash.

The German Merchants made a common practice of adding clary sage and elder flowers to Rhine wine to make it imitate a good Muscatel was so well known that Germans still call the herb Muskateller Salbei and the English know it as Muscatel Sage. Clary sage sometimes replaced hops in beer to produce an enhanced state of intoxication and exhilaration, although this reportedly was often followed by a severe headache. It was considered a 12th century aphrodisiac.

Medicinal Uses

"Like its relative sage, clary tea, the leaf juice in ale or beer, was recommended for many types of women's problems, including delayed or painful menstruation. It was once used to stop night sweating in tuberculosis patients. An astringent is gargled, douched and poured over skin wounds. It is combined with other herbs for kidney problems. The clary seeds form a thick mucilage when soaked for a few minutes and placed in the eye, helps to removed, small irritating particles. A tea of the leaves is also used as an eyewash. Clary is also used to reduce muscle spasms. It is used today mainly to treat digestive problems such as gas and indigestion. It is also regarded as a tonic, calming herb that helps relieve premenstrual problems. *Because of its estrogen-stimulating action, clary sage is most effective when levels of this hormone are low. The plant can therefore be a valuable remedy for complaints associated with menopause, particularly hot flashes.*"

Sclareol

What is Sclareol and why am I discussing it here?

From Wikipedia:

"Sclareol is a fragrant chemical compound found in clary sage (Salvia sclarea), from which it derives its name. It is classified as a bicyclic diterpene alcohol. It is an amber colored solid with a sweet, balsamic scent.[55]

Sclareol is used as a fragrance in cosmetics and perfumes and as flavoring in food. Sclareol and other similar substances may be prepared from sclareolide.

Sclareol is also able to kill human leukemic cells and colon cancer cells by apoptosis.

Sclareol is a phytoestrogen. Is there any proof of this anywhere? PubMed? Research databases? No. Not that I can find. Nothing solid.

The above Wikipedia research indicates it has certain estrogen like anti-cancer benefits. Plust there's a study in Iran which shows it reduces breast cancer risk and cell growth – so does estrodial.

For more information on this subject: please see my book, ***Essential Oils and Healthy Menopause: History and Research Secrets*** available on Amazon and iBooks.

If you enjoyed this book, please leave a review to help others find this information.

Want to Connect With Dr. Purser?

For Dr. Purser's Amazon Author Page linking to all of his books (including his ten #1 books): http://www.greatmedebooks.com

Facebook: Dan Purser MD

Twitter @danpursermd

Pinterest: Dan Purser MD

DanPurserMD.com

© Copyright by Dan Purser MD of Medutainment, Inc.

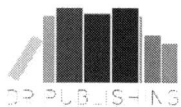

References

[1] No author listed. Accessed 14 August, 2016 online at http://www.physio-pedia.com/Theories_of_Aging.

[2] Hulley S, Grady D, Bush T, et al. Randomized trial of estrogen plus progestin for secondary prevention of
coronary heart disease in postmenopausal women: Heart and Estrogen/progestin Replacement Study
(HERS) Research Group. JAMA 1998;280:605-613.

[3] Grady, D. A New Look at Estrogen and Stroke. 2001 Feb 6. New York Times, pp 1, Health Section.

[4] Hargrove, JT; Eisenberg, E. Menopause. Medical Clinics of North America, Volume 79, Issue 6, 1995, Pages 1337-1356.

[5] [no author listed] Findings from the WHI Postmenopausal Hormone Therapy Trials. Available online at www.nhlbi.nih.gov/whi/. Accessed 2006 Sep 10.

[6] NHLBI Stops Trial of Estrogen Plus Progestin Due to Increased Breast Cancer Risk, Lack of Overall Benefit. NIH News Release, Tuesday, July 9, 2002; pp 1-4.

[7] Berger, L. On Hormone Therapy, The Dust Is Still Settling. 2004 June 6. New York Times, pp 1, Health Section.

[8] Reeves GK, Beral V, et al. Hormonal therapy for menopause and breast-cancer risk by histological type: a cohort study and meta-analysis. Lancet Oncol. 2006 Nov;7(11):910-8.

[9] Genazzani AR, Gambacciani M. The sound of an International anti-HRT herald. Maturitas. 2003 Oct 20;46(2):105-6.

[10] Hulley S, Grady D, Bush T, et al. Randomized trial of estrogen plus progestin for secondary prevention
of coronary heart disease in postmenopausal women: Heart and Estrogen/progestin Replacement Study
(HERS) Research Group. JAMA 1998;280:605-613.

[11] Campagnoli C, Ambroggio S, Biglia N, Sismondi P. Conjugated estrogens and breast cancer risk. Gynecol Endocrinol. 1999 Dec;13 Suppl 6:13-9.

[12] Hargrove, JT; Osteen, KC. An Alternative Method of Hormone Replacement Therapy Using the Natural Sex Steroids. Infertility and Reproductive Medicine Clinics of North America. Volume 6, Number 4, October 1995.

[13] Hargrove, JT; Osteen, KC. An Alternative Method of Hormone Replacement Therapy Using the Natural Sex Steroids. Infertility and Reproductive Medicine Clinics of North America. Volume 6, Number 4, October 1995.

[14] Shimizu Y. [Article in Japanese] [Estrogen: estrone (E1), estradiol (E2), estriol (E3) and estetrol (E4)] Nippon Rinsho. 2005 Aug;63 Suppl 8:425-38.

[15] Hunt CM, Westerkam WR, Stave GM. Effect of age and gender on the activity of human hepatic CYP3A. Biochem Pharmacol 1992;44:275-83.

[16] Robb-Nicholson C. By the way, doctor. In the lead article about HRT use in your April issue, you didn't mention Estrace. I've taken it for several years, without any problems. But am I getting the same benefits as I would with Premarin, and are the risks similar? Harv Womens Health Watch. 2000; 8(2):8 (ISSN: 1070-910X).

[17] Dubey RK, Imthurn B, Barton M, Jackson EK. Vascular consequences of menopause and hormone therapy: importance of timing of treatment and type of estrogen. Cardiovasc Res. 2005 May 1;66(2):295-306.

[18] No author listed. Accessed online on 16 August 2016 at http://worldlinkmedical.com/transdermal-vs-oral-e2-estradiol/

[19] Psaty, BM et al. Hormone Replacement Therapy, Prothrombotic Mutations, and the Risk of Incident Nonfatal Myocardial Infarction in Postmenopausal Women. JAMA. 2001;285:906-913.

[20] Wachter, K. Treat the Very Elderly for Low Bone Density: Bone loss accelerates as patients age, yet
'we aren't doing a very good job' of treating the very elderly. Family Practice News, Volume 35, Issue 9,
Page 67 (01 May 2005).

[21] Siris ES, Miller PD, Barrett-Connor E, Faulkner KG, Wehren LE, Abbott TA, Berger ML, Santora AC,
Sherwood LM. Identification and fracture outcomes of undiagnosed low bone mineral density in
postmenopausal women: results from the National Osteoporosis Risk Assessment. JAMA. 2001 Dec
12;286(22):2815-22.

[22] Davidson, MR. Pharmacotherapeutics for Osteoporosis Prevention and Treatment. J Midwifery Womens
Health 48(1):39-54, 2003. © 2003 Elsevier Science, Inc.

[23] Villareal DT, Binder EF, Williams DB, Schechtman KB, Yarasheski KE, Kohrt WM. Bone mineral
density response to estrogen replacement in frail elderly women: a randomized controlled trial. JAMA.
2001 Aug 15;286(7):815-20.

[24] Sipila S, Heikkinen E, Cheng S, Suominen H, Saari P, Kovanen V, Alen M, Rantanen T. Endogenous
hormones, muscle strength, and risk of fall-related fractures in older women. J Gerontol A Biol Sci Med
Sci. 2006 Jan;61(1):92-6.

[25] Lanham-New SA. Nutritional Influences on Bone Health: An Update

on Current Research and Clinical Implications. [online] Available at www.medscape.com/viewprogram/5034_pnt.

[26] Adams J; Pepping J. Vitamin K in the Treatment and Prevention of Osteoporosis and Arterial Calcification. Am J Health-Syst Pharm. 2005;62(15):1574-1581. ©2005 American Society of Health-System Pharmacists.

[27] Adams J; Pepping J. Vitamin K in the Treatment and Prevention of Osteoporosis and Arterial Calcification. Am J Health-Syst Pharm. 2005;62(15):1574-1581. ©2005 American Society of Health-System Pharmacists.

[28] Cranney A, Wells G, et al; Osteoporosis Methodology Group and The Osteoporosis Research Advisory Group. Meta-analyses of therapies for postmenopausal osteoporosis. II. Meta-analysis of alendronate for the treatment of postmenopausal women. Endocr Rev. 2002 Aug;23(4):508-16.

[29] Davidson, MR. Pharmacotherapeutics for Osteoporosis Prevention and Treatment. J Midwifery Womens Health 48(1):39-54, 2003. © 2003 Elsevier Science, Inc.

[30] Quandt SA, Thompson DE, Schneider DL, Nevitt MC, Black DM. Effect of alendronate on vertebral fracture risk in women with bone mineral density T scores of -1.6 to -2.5 at the femoral neck: the Fracture Intervention Trial. Mayo Clin Proc March 2005;80:343-9.

[31] Schousboe JT, et al. Cost-effectiveness of alendronate therapy for osteopenic postmenopausal women. Ann Intern Med May 3, 2005;142:734-41.

[32] Ference, J.D.; Wilson, S.A. STEPS: Ibandronate (Boniva) for Treatment and Prevention of Osteoporosis in Postmenopausal Women. American Family Physician; January 15, 2006 (table of contents) Vol. 73 No. 2:305-306.

[33] Ference, J.D.; Wilson, S.A. STEPS: Ibandronate (Boniva) for Treatment and Prevention of Osteoporosis in Postmenopausal Women. American Family Physician; January 15, 2006 (table of contents) Vol. 73 No. 2:305-306.

[34] Bischoff-Ferrari HA, Willett WC, Wong JB, Giovannucci E, Dietrich T, Dawson-Hughes B. Fracture prevention with vitamin D supplementation: a meta-analysis of randomized controlled trials. JAMA 2005:293; 2257-64.

[35] Boonen S, Lips P, Bouillon R, Bischoff-Ferrari HA, Vanderschueren D, Haentjens P. Need for additional calcium to reduce the risk of hip fracture with vitamin D supplementation: evidence from a comparative meta-analysis of randomized controlled trials. J Clin Endocrinol Metab. 2007 Jan 30.

[36] Quandt SA; Thompson DE; Schneider DL; Nevitt MC; Black DM.

Effect of alendronate on vertebral fracture risk in women with bone mineral density T scores of-1.6 to -2.5 at the femoral neck: the Fracture Intervention Trial. Mayo Clin Proc. 2005; 80(3):343-9 (ISSN: 0025-6196).

[37] Ishida Y, Kawai S. Comparative efficacy of hormone replacement therapy, etidronate, calcitonin, alfacalcidol, and vitamin K in postmenopausal women with osteoporosis: The Yamaguchi Osteoporosis Prevention Study. Am J Med. 2004 Oct 15;117(8):549-55.

[38] Sipila S, Heikkinen E, Cheng S, Suominen H, Saari P, Kovanen V, Alen M, Rantanen T. Endogenous hormones, muscle strength, and risk of fall-related fractures in older women. J Gerontol A Biol Sci Med Sci. 2006 Jan;61(1):92-6.

[39] Lanham-New SA. Nutritional Influences on Bone Health: An Update on Current Research and Clinical Implications . [online] Available at www.medscape.com/viewprogram/5034_pnt.

[40] Adams J; Pepping J. Vitamin K in the Treatment and Prevention of Osteoporosis and Arterial Calcification. Am J Health-Syst Pharm. 2005;62(15):1574-1581. ©2005 American Society of Health- System Pharmacists.

[41] Ross EA, Szabo NJ, Tebbett IR. Lead content of calcium supplements. JAMA. 2000 Sep 20;284(11):1425-9.

[42] Shah SV; Alam MG. Role of iron in atherosclerosis. Am J Kidney Dis. 2003; 41(3 Suppl 1):S80-3 (ISSN: 1523-6838).

[43] Valko M, Morris H, Cronin MT. Metals, toxicity and oxidative stress. Curr Med Chem. 2005;12(10):1161-208.

[44] New SA. Acid-base homeostasis in the skeleton: Is there a fruit and vegetable link to bone health? In: New SA, Bonjour JP, eds. Nutritional Aspects of Bone Health. Cambridge, UK: Royal Society of Chemistry; 2003: 291-311.

[45] Van Meurs JBJ, Dhonukshe-Rutten RAM, Pluijm SMF, et al. Homocysteine levels and the risk of osteoporotic fracture. N Engl J Med. 2004;350:2033-2041.

[46] Leiblum S, Bachmann GA, Kemmann E, Colburn D, Swartzman L. Vaginal atrophy and the postmenopausal woman: the importance of sexual activity and hormones. JAMA 1983;249:2195-8.

[47] Kightlinger, RS. Menopause Matters. Vaginal Atrophy: Clinical Evaluation and Management. Available online at http://www.femalepatient.com/html/arc/sig/meno/articles/030_04_065.asp. Accessed March 19, 2007.

[48] Cobin, Rh. HRT and Cardiocascular Protection (January 2001 -- Live Event). Medical Crossfire, June 2001; Vol. 3 [6]: 139-40.

[49] Psaty, BM et al. Hormone Replacement Therapy, Prothrombotic Mutations, and the Risk of Incident Nonfatal Myocardial Infarction in Postmenopausal Women. JAMA. 2001;285:906-913.

[50] Campagnoli C; Colombo P; De Aloysio D; Gambacciani M; Grazioli I; Nappi C; Serra GB; Genazzani AR. Positive effects on cardiovascular and breast metabolic markers of oral estradiol and dydrogesterone in comparison with transdermal estradiol and norethisterone acetate. Maturitas. 2002; 41(4):299-311 (ISSN: 0378-5122).

[51] Bastian LA, Smith CM, Nanda K. Is this woman perimenopausal? JAMA. 2003 Feb 19;289(7):895-902.

[52] Dalal, S; Zhukovsky, DS. Pathoilable online at physiology and Management of Hot Flashes. www.SupportiveOncology.net; VOLUME 4, NUMBER 7; JULY/AUGUST 2006. Available online at www.SupportiveOncology.net.

[53] Freedman RR, Norton D, Woodward S, et al. Core body temperature and circadian rhythm of hot flashes in menopausal women. J Clin Endocrinol Metab 1995;80:2354–2358.

[54] Cho JJ, Cadet P, Salamon E, Mantione K, Stefano GB. The nongenomic protective effects of estrogen on the male cardiovascular system: clinical and therapeutic implications in aging men. Med Sci Monit. 2003 Mar;9(3):RA63-8.

[55] No author listed. Accessed 31 May 2015 online at http://www.thegoodscentscompany.com/data/rw1018631.html

Made in the USA
Middletown, DE
16 July 2018